STRETCH EXERCISE FOR SENIORS

Essential Stretching Exercises Tailored for Vibrant Seniors To Relief Pain, Stress, Joint health, Improve Balance, Strength, and Improve Posture

Dr. LANDON STONE

Table of Contents

CHAPTER ONE

Unlocking the Benefits of Stretching for Active Senior Living

Maintaining an active and healthy lifestyle becomes increasingly important as we age gracefully. The skill of stretching is a powerful and easily available instrument in this pursuit. In this section, we will look at the critical role that stretching plays in the well-being of seniors, revealing a world of benefits that go far beyond basic flexibility.

Understanding the Importance of Senior Stretching

As we age, our bodies go through natural changes that affect our flexibility, joint health, and general physical comfort. Many daily tasks are sedentary, and the gradual loss of muscle mass can contribute to stiffness, restricted range of motion, and greater susceptibility to joint pain. Stretching emerges as a critical ally in overcoming these obstacles.

The Most Important Advantages of Stretching for Senior Health

1 .One of the key benefits of frequent stretching for seniors is the potential to relieve discomfort, particularly in the joints and muscles. Gentle stretching exercises aid in the improvement of circulation, the reduction of inflammation, and the release of endorphins, the body's natural pain relievers.

2. Stress Reduction: Seniors frequently confront a variety of pressures, ranging from health difficulties to lifestyle changes. Stretching not only provides physical relief, but it also functions as a conscious practice. Stretching with controlled, focused motions can assist to quiet the mind, lowering tension and increasing mental well-being.

3. Joint Health: It is critical for elders to maintain healthy joints, and stretching can help them do so. Stretching activities improve joint function by increasing flexibility and lubricating the joints, lowering the likelihood of stiffness and discomfort.

4. Balance Improvement: Falls are a major worry for seniors, frequently resulting in injuries

that limit independence. Balance and coordination stretching activities assist seniors build stability, reducing the risk of falls and improving overall mobility.

5. Stretching is commonly associated with flexibility, but it also helps to muscle strength. Incorporating resistance into stretching exercises aids in muscle maintenance and growth, encouraging an active and vibrant lifestyle.

6. Posture Support: Age-related changes in posture can result in problems such as slouching or hunching. Stretching exercises that target core muscles and the spine can considerably improve posture while also improving overall physical attractiveness and comfort.

We go on a journey to appreciate the full potential of this simple yet transforming activity by understanding the enormous influence of stretching on senior health. Throughout this guide, we will look at customized stretching routines, balance-enhancing exercises, strength-building strategies, and other techniques to help seniors live lives of flexibility, vitality, and long-term well-being.

Seniors' Common Health Issues

Our bodies change as we age, and these changes can have an influence on our health. To maintain a high quality of life, it is critical to recognize and address these difficulties. Seniors may experience the following health issues:

1.   Reduced   Flexibility: Aging frequently causes a natural decline in   flexibility,   making   daily activities more difficult and raising the risk of injury.

2. Joint Stiffness: Seniors may have joint stiffness due to a decrease   in   synovial   fluid production and cartilage wear and tear.

3. Sarcopenia, or the age-related decrease of muscle mass, can cause weakness, limited mobility, and an increased risk of falling.

4. Chronic Pain: Conditions such as   arthritis   and   other   chronic illnesses can contribute to chronic pain, affecting overall comfort and mobility.

5. Limited Range of Motion: As elders age, their ability to move

freely and comfortably may deteriorate, affecting the ease with which they undertake daily activities.

Stretching Helps with Pain, Stress, and Joint Health

Stretching appears as a diverse answer to the following typical health issues encountered by seniors:

1. Pain Relief: Gentle stretching exercises stimulate blood flow to the muscles and joints, relieving tension and pain. Stretching activities on a regular basis can be an important part of a pain treatment approach.

2. Stress Reduction: Physical discomfort is frequently exacerbated by stress. Stretching not only benefits the body, but it

also has a mindfulness component that aids in stress reduction through focused, intentional motions and controlled breathing.

3. Joint Lubrication: Stretching stimulates the production of synovial fluid, which lubricates and stretches the joints. This is especially good for elders who have joint stiffness or soreness.

4. Stretching actively works to enhance flexibility and range of motion, combating the natural deterioration associated with aging. As a result, elders can preserve their independence and do everyday duties more easily.

5. Muscle Activation: Stretching exercises engage and activate muscles, preventing muscle atrophy and increasing overall strength.

The Value of Exercise for Seniors

A commitment to regular exercise, in addition to targeted stretching, is vital for senior well-being. Exercise has various advantages, including:

1. Aerobic workouts promote cardiovascular health, circulation, and stamina.

2. Weight-bearing workouts help to preserve bone density, which lowers the risk of osteoporosis.

3. Physical activity releases endorphins, which promotes a pleasant mood and lowers the risk of depression and anxiety.

4. Maintaining Independence: Regular exercise, especially stretching, helps seniors keep their

independence and actively participate in daily life.

Individuals can engage on a journey toward greater well-being, flexibility, and vitality by recognizing the specific health concerns elders encounter and the role stretching plays in treating them. In the following chapters, we will look at customized stretching routines developed to meet the specific needs of seniors.

Starting Out Safely

Seniors must emphasize safety before beginning a stretching and exercise routine. This tutorial is dedicated to providing a thorough overview of how to begin a stretching program properly. This chapter attempts to build the groundwork for a safe and beneficial senior fitness journey by emphasizing the value of pre-exercise assessments, emphasizing the importance of consulting healthcare specialists, and combining efficient warm-up and cool-down procedures.

Seniors' Pre-Exercise Evaluation

Seniors must undertake a pre-exercise assessment before engaging in any physical activity. This examination assists people in understanding their present fitness level, identifying potential risks, and tailoring their training regimen accordingly. A pre-exercise assessment should include the following elements:

1. Health History: Keeping track of any existing medical illnesses, injuries, or surgeries can provide significant insight into potential

restrictions or areas that require special attention.

2. Assessing current range of motion, joint flexibility, and general mobility allows you to personalize stretching exercises to your specific needs.

3. Understanding baseline strength and endurance levels aids in determining the optimum intensity of exercises and ensuring progressive progression.

4. Assessing balance and coordination can help suggest workouts that can improve stability and lower the chance of falling.

5. Identifying any current pain or discomfort allows for activity modifications to avoid exacerbating difficulties and

promotes a safe and enjoyable training experience.

Consultation with Healthcare Professionals is Critical

Consultation with healthcare specialists, such as physicians or physical therapists, is an important step in ensuring the safety and efficacy of a senior's exercise plan. Important considerations include:

1. Medical clearance: Obtaining medical clearance allows you to identify any contraindications or specific measures that should be taken based on your health state.

2. Exercise Tailoring: Healthcare experts can make individualized recommendations and changes to accommodate existing health issues or concerns.

3. Medication Monitoring: Some drugs may have an effect on exercise tolerance or interact with certain activities. Healthcare professionals can advise you on how to modify your training routine accordingly.

4. Addressing Concerns: Seniors can talk to healthcare experts about any concerns, fears, or uncertainties they have about starting an exercise program, promoting a sense of confidence and reassurance.

Seniors' Warm-Up and Cool-Down Techniques

Warm-up and cool-down routines are critical components of any workout program, especially for seniors. These strategies prepare the body for action, reduce injury risk, and enhance flexibility:

1. Warm-Up:

• Cardiovascular Warm-Up: Aerobic activities such as brisk walking or stationary cycling raise heart rate and blood flow.

• Joint Mobilization: Gently moving key joints prepares them for greater ranges of motion during stretching activities.

• Dynamic Stretching: Including dynamic stretches in your routine, such as leg swings or arm circles, gradually enhances flexibility and warms up muscles.

2. Cool-Down:

• Static Stretching: Holding modest stretches for each major muscle group aids in the prevention of stiffness and increases flexibility.

• Deep Breathing: Deep, controlled breathing improves relaxation and aids in progressively lowering heart rate.

• Hydration: Keeping hydrated during and after exercise benefits general health and recovery.

Seniors can begin their stretching and exercise routine with confidence by emphasizing the importance of pre-exercise assessments, consulting healthcare professionals, and incorporating warm-up and cool-down techniques, reducing the risk of injury and maximizing the benefits of their fitness journey.

CHAPTER TWO

Stretching Routines Customized

We get right to the heart of your stretching journey by presenting senior-specific stretching practices. Each section focuses on a different part of the body, with simple directions and explanations for four main areas: neck and shoulder stretches, back and spine stretches, hip and leg stretches, and arm and wrist stretches.

Stretches for the Neck and Shoulders

❖ Neck Rolling:

1. Sit or stand up straight, with your spine straight.

2. Tilt your head slowly to one side, bringing your ear near your shoulder.

3. Roll your neck forward and then to the opposing side gently.

4. Repeat in both directions, moving slowly and deliberately.

5. This stretch improves neck flexibility and relieves shoulder stress.

> ❖ **Squeeze of the Shoulder Blades:**

1. Sit or stand with good posture and relaxed shoulders.

2. Squeeze your shoulder blades together as if holding a pencil between them.

3. Squeeze for 5-10 seconds and then release.

4. Repeat for a total of 10-15 times.

5. This stretch focuses on the upper back and improves posture.

Stretching of the Back and Spine

➢ Forward Bend While Seated:

1. Place your feet flat on the floor and sit on the edge of a chair.

2. Inhale, stretch your spine, and exhale while hingeing at the hips and reaching for your toes.

3. Hold the stretch for 15-30 seconds, allowing your spine and hamstrings to relax.

4. Return to an upright position gradually.

5. This stretch improves lower back and hamstring flexibility.

➢ **Stretching the Cat-Cow:**

1. Begin in a tabletop position on your hands and knees.

2. Inhale deeply, arch your back, and raise your head and tailbone to the ceiling (Cow).

3. Exhale, circle your back, and tuck your chin in (Cat).

4. Repeat the preceding steps for 1-2 minutes.

5. This stretch improves flexibility and mobility across the spine.

Leg and hip stretches

o **Hip opener while seated:**

1. Sit up straight with your back straight and your feet flat on the floor.

2. One ankle should be crossed over the opposing knee.

3. Gently press down on the crossed knee, feeling the hip stretch.

4. Hold for 15 to 30 seconds before switching sides.

5. This stretch focuses on the hips and improves hip flexibility.

- o Stretch your quadriceps while standing.

1. Place your feet hip-width apart.

2. Bend one knee and put your heel to your buttocks.

3. Hold your ankle with one hand and feel the stretch at the front of your thigh.

4. Hold for 15 to 30 seconds before switching sides.

5. This stretch focuses on the quadriceps and improves leg flexibility.

Wrist and arm stretches

❖ Stretching the Wrist Flexors:

1. Extend one arm out in front of you, palm down.

2. Gently press down on the fingers with the opposite hand.

3. Hold for 15 to 30 seconds before switching sides.

4. This stretch focuses on the flexors of the forearm and wrist.

❖ Triceps Extension:

1. Raise one arm above your head, bend your elbow, and reach your hand down your back.

2. Gently push on the bent elbow with your opposing hand.

3. Hold for 15 to 30 seconds before switching sides.

4. This stretch primarily works the triceps and upper arms.

By implementing these individualized stretching routines into your daily routine, you will not only improve flexibility but also relieve tension, improve joint health, and promote general well-being. Remember to breathe deeply and comfortably throughout the movements and to do each stretch in a controlled manner. Improving Coordination and Balance

Maintaining and improving balance and coordination becomes increasingly important as we age in order to maintain independence and avoid falls. This chapter presents exercises intended specifically for seniors to improve balance and coordination. By implementing these routines into your routine, you not only improve your stability but also your physical confidence and well-being.

Exercises to Improve Balance

> **Stand with a single leg:**

1. If necessary, stand near a firm surface for support.

2. Lift one foot off the ground while remaining balanced on the other.

3. Hold the position for 10-30 seconds.

4. Repeat with the other legs.

5. Do 2-3 sets on each leg.

6. This exercise strengthens the muscles that control balance.

> **Walk from heel to toe:**

1. Place one foot's heel precisely in front of the other foot's toes.

2. Walk in a straight line, with the heel of one foot directly in front of the toes of the other.

3. Maintain a straight path and a steady speed.

4. Continue for a total of 20 steps.

5. This workout enhances your balance and coordination.

Seniors' Coordination and Stability Exercises

o **Marching in Time:**

1. Place your feet hip-width apart.

2. March in place by raising your knees to your chest.

3. Swing your arms in a synchronized motion.

4. Continue for another 1-2 minutes.

5. This exercise improves coordination and balance.

o **Raises on the side legs:**

1. Place your feet hip-width apart.

2. Lift one leg straight out to the side.

3. Return to your starting point.

4. Rep with the other leg.

5. Repeat 10-15 times on each side.

6. This exercise strengthens the hip abductors and improves stability.

Stretching's Role in Balance Improvement

Stretching, in addition to focused balance exercises, plays an important role in improving overall balance and stability in seniors:

❖ Leg Swings with Dynamic Motion:

1. For stability, place yourself near a stable surface.

2. Swing one leg forward and backward with control.

3. Swing each leg 10-15 times.

4. Change to swinging the leg from side to side.

5. This dynamic stretching exercise increases flexibility and helps with balance.

❖ **Tree Pose in Yoga:**

1. Place your feet hip-width apart.

2. Place your weight on one foot.

3. Place the opposite foot's sole against the inner thigh or calf.

4. Gather your palms in front of your chest.

5. Maintain the posture for 15-30 seconds.

6. Repeat with the other legs.

7. This yoga pose incorporates stretching and balance improvement.

By implementing these balance and coordination exercises into your everyday routine, along with targeted stretching routines, you actively contribute to maintaining and enhancing your general stability. Regular practice builds movement confidence, lowers the danger of falling, and improves your ability to navigate daily activities with ease. Remember to execute these exercises at your own pace and intensity, and to contact with healthcare professionals if you have any concerns or specific health conditions.

Senior Strengthening Exercises

Strength is an essential component of general well-being, especially as we age. This chapter provides customized strengthening exercises for seniors, with an emphasis on incorporating resistance into stretching regimens. Incorporating targeted strength-building stretches not only improves muscular tone but also fortifies your body against the effects of aging. Furthermore, we'll look at the several advantages of integrating stretching and strength training in a holistic fitness strategy.

Resistance in Stretching

> **Squats with a Resistance Band:**

1. Place a resistance band directly above your knees.

2. Step on the band with your feet shoulder-width apart.

3. Squat down, keeping your knees aligned with your toes.

4. Return to your starting point.

5. Complete 2-3 sets of 10-15 repetitions.

6. The quadriceps, hamstrings, and glutes are worked on in this workout.

> **Leg Press with a Stability Ball:**

1. Place a stability ball against a wall and sit.

2. Press your feet shoulder-width apart against the wall.

3. Lift your hips off the ball by extending your legs.

4. Return to the beginning posture by bending your knees.

5. Complete 2-3 sets of 10-12 repetitions.

6. This exercise works on quadriceps strength and leg stability.

Stretches to Increase Strength

❖ **Squats in a Chair with an Overhead Reach:**

1. Face a sturdy chair with your feet shoulder-width apart.

2. Squat down and extend your arms forward.

3. Stand up again and extend your arms overhead.

4. Complete 2-3 sets of 12-15 repetitions.

5. This workout strengthens the lower body while also improving general strength.

❖ **Push-ups against the wall:**

1. Face a wall with your arms extended at shoulder height.

2. Perform push-ups against the wall by leaning forward.

3. Complete 2-3 sets of 10-15 repetitions.

4. This workout works on chest, shoulders, and triceps strength.

The Advantages of Using Stretching and Strength Training Together

1. Stretching and strength exercise together improves general flexibility, lowering the risk of injury and promoting a greater range of motion.

2. Strengthening exercises help with muscle control and coordination, which improves general stability and balance.

3. Weight-bearing workouts combined with stretching boost

bone health, lowering the incidence of osteoporosis and fractures.

4. Strength exercise, when paired with stretching, promotes joint health by improving appropriate alignment and minimizing joint tension.

5. Efficient Caloric Burn: A well-rounded workout routine that combines stretching and strength training promotes weight loss and enhances overall energy expenditure.

6. Endurance and Muscle Tone: Including resistance in stretching practices helps build and maintain muscle tone, which contributes to enhanced endurance and stamina.

7. Functional fitness is enhanced by strengthening workouts that

mirror daily activities, making it simpler to do actions like lifting, reaching, and bending with ease.

By incorporating targeted strength-building stretches and incorporating resistance into stretching regimens, you go on a road toward a more robust, toned, and functional body. Stretching and strength training work together to provide a holistic approach to senior fitness, ensuring that you not only maintain but actively increase your physical well-being. Before beginning a new fitness plan, always contact with a healthcare practitioner, especially if you have any pre-existing health ailments or concerns.

CHAPTER THREE

Posture Improvement

Maintaining excellent posture is an important facet of general health, especially as we age. This part discusses the effects of aging on posture, includes stretching exercises intended expressly for posture improvement, and offers practical ergonomic advice to encourage improved posture in daily activities.

The Influence of Aging on Posture

Various factors contribute to changes in posture as we age. These are some examples:

1. Muscle Weakness: As we age, natural muscle loss can weaken the support framework for the

spine, resulting in a stooped or slumped posture.

2. Changes in Bone Density: Aging-related bone density loss can lead to changes in spinal alignment.

3. Joint Stiffness: Joint stiffness, particularly in the spine, can impair mobility and lead to poor posture.

4. Reduced Flexibility: Lack of flexibility can lead to limits in range of motion, impairing one's ability to maintain good posture.

Stretching to Improve Posture

Incorporating targeted stretches into your regimen can assist in mitigating the effects of aging on posture:

> **Stretch for Thoracic Extension:**

1. Maintain a straight spine while sitting or standing.

2. Put your hands behind your back.

3. Arch your upper back gently backward, expanding your chest.

4. Hold for 15-30 seconds, allowing your upper back to stretch.

5. Repeat 2-3 times more.

> **The Child's Pose:**

1. Begin by getting down on your hands and knees.

2. Sit back on your heels, arms extended front.

3. Maintain a stretch in your lower back and shoulders by keeping your spine extended.

4. Maintain for 30 seconds to 1 minute.

5. Repeat as necessary.

Ergonomic Suggestions for Improved Posture in Daily Activities

1. Keep a Neutral Spine at Work:

• Adjust your chair and computer monitor to keep your spine in a neutral position while sitting.

• Take frequent breaks to stretch, stand, and move around.

2. Exercise Good Body Mechanics:

• When lifting objects, bend at the hips and knees rather than the waist.

• Avoid heavy lifting and repetitive back-stretching activities.

3. Invest in Helpful Furniture:

• Select a mattress and pillows that provide adequate spinal support when sleeping.

• Sit on supportive chairs that promote healthy posture.

4. Keep Screen Time in Mind:

• Keep screens at eye level to avoid neck and upper back strain.

• Take breaks from long periods of screen time to stretch and change postures.

5. Including Posture Exercises in Your Routine:

• Incorporate posture-focused workouts into your normal training regimen.

• Build core strength to support the spine and keep it in optimal position.

6. Standing and Sitting with Awareness:

• When sitting, maintain your weight properly distributed on both hips and your feet flat on the floor.

• Stand shoulder-width apart with your feet shoulder-width apart, shoulders back, and chin parallel to the ground.

7. Stretching breaks should be taken on a regular basis.

• Throughout the day, take short breaks to stretch and reset your posture.

• Include moderate stretches that target areas of stress.

You can actively work towards developing and maintaining excellent posture by recognizing the influence of aging on posture, performing targeted stretching exercises, and incorporating ergonomic advice into daily tasks. These practices not only lead to a more confident and upright appearance, but also to a healthier and more comfortable general well-being. Before beginning new exercises, always contact with a healthcare practitioner, especially if you have any pre-existing health ailments or concerns.

Creating a Reliable Routine

Developing and sticking to a stretching regimen is critical for enjoying the long-term advantages of increased flexibility, strength, and overall well-being. This section will walk novices through the process of developing a realistic and feasible stretching program. It also gives seniors incentive to continue active and techniques for overcoming obstacles and staying dedicated to their fitness goal.

Developing a Realistic and Doable Stretching Routine

1. Begin slowly: Begin with a few simple stretches and progressively add more as time goes on. Avoid overexertion and pay attention to your body's signals.

2. Establish a Routine: Schedule your stretching routine for specified times of the day. This could be done in the morning to get you going for the day or in the evening to unwind.

3. Set Realistic Goals: Establish specific and attainable goals for your stretching program. Having defined goals, whether it's improving flexibility, lowering discomfort, or better balance, keeps you motivated.

4. Include a range of stretches to target various muscle groups and components of fitness. This gives variation to your routine and keeps you from becoming bored.

5. Adapt to Your Comfort Level: Modify stretches according to your level of comfort. It is critical to experience a slight stretch without

experiencing pain. Adjust or skip any stretches that seem uncomfortable.

Tips to Motivate Seniors to Stay Active

1. Appreciate minor Wins: Recognize and appreciate your progress, no matter how minor. Every step toward a healthier living is a victory.

2. Make it Fun: Select stretches and exercises that you enjoy. Make your practice pleasurable by listening to music, practicing in a scenic location, or doing it with a friend.

3. keep Socially linked: To keep socially linked, join group classes, clubs, or fitness communities. Motivation and support can be provided via companionship and shared goals.

4. Visualize Your Goals: Visualize the wonderful outcomes you wish to attain from your stretching regimen. Visualization can be a very effective motivator.

5. Reward Yourself: When you reach certain milestones in your routine, treat yourself to a modest reward. This can serve as a motivator to continue your efforts.

Overcoming Obstacles and Remaining Committed

1. Address Physical limits: Consult with healthcare providers to adapt your routine if you have physical limits or health issues. They can advise on safe and effective exercises.

2. Create a Routine: Consistency is essential. Make stretching a regular part of your daily or

weekly calendar by scheduling it at specified times.

3. Accountability Partner: Enlist the help of a friend or family member in your stretching routine. Having someone to accompany you on your path improves accountability and inspiration.

4. Adapt to Changes: Life is fluid, and circumstances can shift. Be flexible in adapting your routine to new situations while being consistent.

5. Incorporate Variety: Keep your routine interesting by incorporating different stretches or activities. This keeps things exciting and fresh.

6. Keep a record of your stretches, noting changes in flexibility,

balance, or any other goals you've set for yourself. Progress tracking can enhance motivation.

Developing a consistent stretching routine takes time and effort, but the benefits in terms of increased health and well-being are enormous. Seniors can embark on a road of enduring fitness and vitality by setting realistic goals, staying inspired, and conquering obstacles. Before beginning new exercises, always contact with a healthcare practitioner, especially if you have any pre-existing health ailments or concerns.

Conclusion

Motivation to Live a Healthier and More Active Lifestyle

As we come to the end of this thorough guide on stretching

exercises for seniors, it's critical to reinforce the powerful path you've made toward a healthier, more active lifestyle. Your dedication to integrate stretching, balance exercises, strength training, and posture improvement into your daily routine is admirable, and it holds the key to achieving revolutionary changes in your health.

Celebrate Your Progress: Take a time to reflect on your accomplishments, no matter how minor. Celebrate each step forward in your fitness quest as proof of your commitment and perseverance. Every stretch, every strengthening activity, and every conscious posture correction helps to improve your overall health.

Embrace the beneficial Changes: As you progress down this road, take attention to the beneficial changes that occur in your body and mind. Take note of the increased flexibility, improved balance, and newfound strength. Enjoy the better posture that not only improves your physical look but also gives you a sense of confidence and well-being.

A Journey, Not a goal: Remember that living a healthier and more active lifestyle is a journey, not a goal. Every day is an opportunity to expand on the foundation you've established by trying new stretches, adding resistance to your workouts, and regularly practicing proper posture.

Recognize the intimate link that exists between your mind and body. The attention you bring to your stretching routines, the conscious focus on balance exercises, and your commitment to strengthening benefits not only your physical health but also your emotional well-being. The tranquility and clarity that come with a more active lifestyle add to a sense of overall fulfillment.

Stay Inspired: Draw motivation from your personal progress as well as the stories of others who have taken similar paths. Whether it's conquering obstacles, reaching fitness milestones, or enjoying unexpected joys along the way, let these stories inspire you to keep active and healthy.

Community and Support: Surround yourself with a positive community, whether it's friends, family, or other fitness aficionados. Share your accomplishments, seek counsel when faced with adversity, and draw strength from the collective energy of individuals who have traveled similar routes.

Your Health, Your Investment: Keep in mind that one of the most precious investments you can make is in your health. The advantages of leading an active lifestyle go far beyond the physical realm, influencing your mental and emotional well-being and, eventually, improving your overall quality of life.

In closing this book, I want to express my heartfelt encouragement to keep embracing the great changes you've started. May your journey to a better, more active lifestyle be filled with joy, resilience, and the contentment that comes from taking control of your health. Here's to the more vibrant and empowered version of yourself in the next days, months, and years. Continue stretching, moving, and thriving!

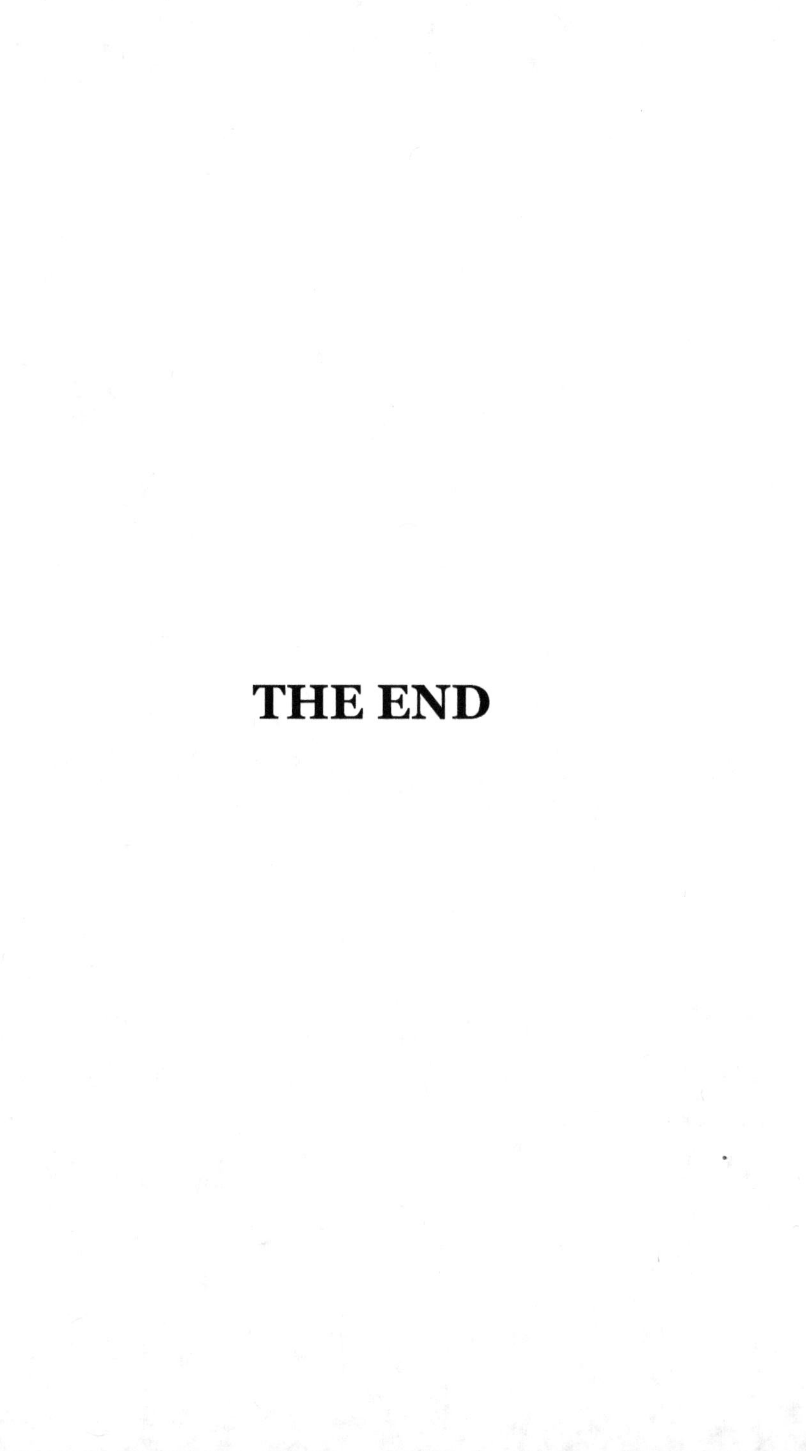

THE END

www.ingramcontent.com/pod-product-compliance
Lightning Source LLC
Chambersburg PA
CBHW071111260726
48661CB00006B/2572